I0439764

NATURAL REMEDIES

Overcome Anxiety, Panic Attacks, Colds and Flu, Menopause, Inflammation & More Natural Cures

Table of Contents

Copyright

Copyright 2015 by Dagny Walters all rights reserved.

This document is geared towards providing exact and reliable information in regards to the topic and issue covered. The publication is sold with the idea that the publisher is not required to render accounting, officially permitted, or otherwise, qualified services. If advice is necessary, legal or professional, a practiced individual in the profession should be ordered.

- From a Declaration of Principles which was accepted and approved equally by a Committee of the American Bar Association and a Committee of Publishers and Associations.

In no way is it legal to reproduce, duplicate, or transmit any part of this document in either electronic means or in printed format. Recording of this publication is strictly prohibited and any storage of this document is not allowed unless with written permission from the publisher. All rights reserved.

The information provided herein is stated to be truthful and consistent, in that any liability, in terms of inattention or otherwise, by any usage or abuse of any policies, processes, or directions contained within is the solitary and utter responsibility of the recipient reader. Under no circumstances will any legal responsibility or blame be held against the publisher for any reparation, damages, or monetary loss due to the information herein, either directly or indirectly.

Respective authors own all copyrights not held by the publisher.

The information herein is offered for informational purposes solely, and is universal as so. The presentation of the information is without contract or any type of guarantee assurance.

The trademarks that are used are without any consent, and the publication of the trademark is without permission or backing by the trademark owner. All trademarks and brands within this book are for clarifying purposes only and are the owned by the owners themselves, not affiliated with this document.

Introduction

I want to thank you and congratulate you for purchasing this book, "Natural Remedies: Overcome Anxiety, Panic Attacks, Colds and Flu, Menopause, Inflammation & More - Natural Cures".

This book contains helpful information about different natural cures and their many uses when it comes to healing both mind, and body.

This book will provide you the steps and strategies required to successfully practice homeopathic therapy using ingredients that can be found in your garden!

Chapter 1: What You Need To Know About Herbal Remedies

There are people who quickly dismiss the healing abilities of natural remedies as no more than quackery. However, this is certainly not the case. The use of different botanicals when it comes to curing illnesses and diseases goes back to ancient medical practice. In fact, there is quite a bit of literature on this particular subject and it forms the foundation for many homeopathic medical treatments.

Were you aware that at least a quarter of the medications available today actually contain active ingredients which were derived from known healing plants?

Currently, it is estimated that at least 80% of the population of the world make use of herbs and various other botanicals as a primary source of health care. Worthy of mention would be the different dietary supplements widely available today which all contain powdered or liquid versions of potent herbs such as: garlic, ginseng, echinacea, goldenseal, saw palmetto, ginkgo, ephedra, aloe and cranberry to mention a few.

There are clinical studies being conducted to learn more about healing herbs and other plans in order to make sure that people have a better understanding of its benefits as well as possible side effects. It is important, of course, to develop knowledge of the precautions that users must take and how to properly use a particular herb. Considering that they are quite potent and there are certain side effects such as allergic reactions that can occur if these were to be used mindlessly.

The Advantages

- Herbal remedies are actually much cheaper when compared to more conventional medicines. It is something that everyone would be able to afford and even grow in their own backyards, hence significantly reducing the amount of money they need to shell out. After all, medication these days isn't cheap and many people would often choose to just skip on taking it simply because they cannot afford it.

- Herbal medicines can be taken without the need for a prescription. Some people would still approach a holistic healer and ask for advice but beyond that? You can buy these very easily from your local pharmacy or natural remedy store.

- Herbal medicines, though often overlooked by many, are actually known to be more potent when it comes to other types of medication. If they are completely natural and used in the proper manner as well as for the right purpose, it can certainly help in a big way. In fact, adding chemical components to it can weaken its overall effects.

- The side effects are very minor. In fact, it's only the allergic reactions that people need to be careful with. As long as the herbal medicine is prepared properly and used for the appropriate purpose, it should work without any issues. It should also be noted that natural remedies tend to offer more lasting effects when it comes to a person's overall wellness.

- Herbal medicine can be used to treat obesity safely. In many countries, this particular problem is continuously growing and places a great burden on the individual's own health. Whilst there are medicines already available for treating it, its constant use can actually cause more damage than good. An herbal remedy, on the other hand, can help treat the problem without adding to it.

The Disadvantages

- There are instances wherein herbal medicines are simply not enough and may prove ineffective when it comes to treating more serious ailments. They can be used as supplements but in certain situations, turning to conventional medicine is the more viable solution.

- Because they're more subtle (but not less effective), herbal medication may take longer when it comes to curing certain ailments when compared to conventional medicine. Patience is needed and of course, its use would depend on the needs of the patients themselves. If there's a need for urgent treatment then using conventional medication might be the better option. For this, consult your doctor and ask how you may be able to use herbal remedies as a means of counteracting the negative effects that your current medication has on your body.

• Some people may not be able to use herbal medications due to their allergies. Because there's no prescription needed, any individual who is seeking to use natural remedies to treat themselves should be well aware of their own allergies. Doing a test is possible too but make sure that it is done properly. Conventional medication can cause allergic reactions too but since many of them are prescribed, proper tests can be done prior to prescribing it to a patient.

• Many governments and health care systems do not approve of herbal medication. For the most part, they are taken upon the individual's own risk. There are popular and branded herbal supplements available but even these should be taken with some proper precaution and care. It always pays to do a bit of research before starting your treatment.

- The effects of herbal remedies can actually interact with that of conventional medicine if they are used at the same time. It can heighten the effects or counteract negatives but at the same time, it can turn the properties of the medication toxic and dangerous to consumer. As such, it is best to inform your doctor if you're planning on using herbal medication whilst currently taking a prescription medicine.

Active Ingredients of Medicinal Herbs

Typically, conventional medicine would isolate a single active ingredient that's the most potent for the purpose it is needed for. On the other hand, herbal remedies can have multiple ones and be equally effective. It is not unusual for herbalists to recommend two to three different herbs together to be used in combination in order to achieve a better effect. So if you're planning on trying out natural treatments for yourself, always speak with an herbalist or a natural medicine practitioner. They should be able to help with choosing the right herbs for your needs as well as the right amount to take.

Chapter 2: Remedies for Overcoming Anxiety

There are a number of different prescription medicines available for people who might be experiencing anxiety and panic attacks. These do offer a quick solution and relief from the problem but when it comes to finding a long term solution for the problem, this might not be the right route to take. Ask yourself, do you want to keep on taking the medication indefinitely? If the answer is NO then you might want look at natural alternatives that could help you deal with the anxiety whilst offering you a more long term solution for it.

These natural remedies are better than prescription drugs in certain respects. For example, they are not as strong, which means you're not risking damage to any of your internal organs. Did you know that continuously taking prescribed medicine can actually create subtle changes to the chemical makeup of your body? Herbal remedies are also not addictive so you're not risking becoming dependent on it to feel better. They don't have any major side effects or make you feel withdrawal symptoms once you stop using them. That alone is a massive advantage when you consider modern anxiety medications such as benzodiazepines which can be habit-forming.

Another advantage to using herbal remedies would be the fact that they don't affect your moods unlike other anti-anxiety medication. You won't feel drowsy and lethargic for the rest of the day after taking it. Because they aren't as strong, your reaction time remains the same and you won't feel sluggish. After all, how are you supposed to enjoy the benefits of the treatment if all you want to do is lie in bed after taking it?

Eager to give herbal remedies a try to help with treating anxiety? Here's a shortlist of the most commonly used herbs for this purpose. Just remember to check with your doctor before using any of them to make sure that you're not allergic.

Kava Kava Root

The roots of the Kava plant are often used to make a kind of tea that contains both anesthetic and sedative effects. It is commonly used throughout places such as Polynesia, Vanuatu, Hawaii and even some parts of Micronesia. Studies have also shown that it can be a pretty potent alternative when it comes to treating chronic clinical anxiety as well as panic attacks. There is a lower risk of dependency and an even lower potential for any side effects. There is a proper dosage for this so do ask your physician or a natural medicine doctor for advice on how to use it for yourself.

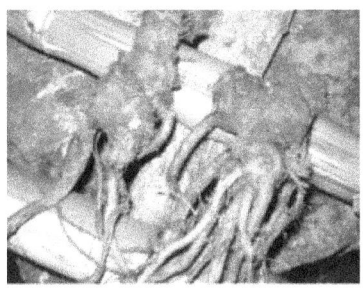

Valerian Root

This particular herb is well known for its relaxing effect and is primarily used to help with promoting better sleep. It is typically given to people who suffer from insomnia as it helps them fall asleep easier but without risking addiction. This same calming effect can also be used to ease anxiety as well as stress. It can relax both the mind and body quite easily. Some people combine its use with meditation or any other form of exercise such as yoga. It has no major side effects but do avoid taking it together with alcohol.

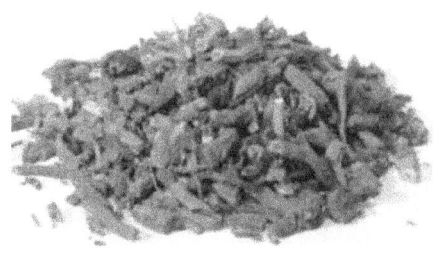

Passion Flower

Its effects are similar to the Kava but more subtle. Research has proven that it can help with relieving moderate anxiety. This means that you have a gentler alternative when it comes to dealing with the issue instead of going with the more potent option. This is great for simple stress relief as well. If you're looking to relax after a long day but the tension won't seem to leave your mind and body- just take some of this and it would help you feel calmer without the sleepiness.

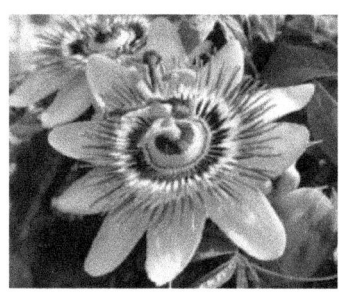

St. John's Wort

This particular herb has been in use for treating mental health issues for hundreds of years now. For people who are suffering from depression, this can provide them with relief- the same goes for individuals who might be dealing with panic attacks and chronic clinical anxiety. It is capable of relaxing the mind and relieving any tension in the body. For insomniacs, it can help with promoting easy sleep. Given that it is a natural remedy, there is no risk of addiction.

Chapter 3: Remedies for Treating Cold & Flu

Treating the symptoms of both the cold and flu can be as simple as popping a pill and getting on with what you need to do. This method works fine but what if there's a much healthier and more affordable option? Try herbal remedies for a change. They are easy to get and prepare. In taking them, you're not bombarding your body with synthetic chemicals which can be more damaging that you first thought. Of course, there's also the added bonus that many of these herbs are actually beneficial to your good health. Here are some of the most effective herbal treatments when it comes to treating the cold and flu:

Thyme

This particular herb is a known expectorant which helps with dry cough and clearing out the lungs quickly. It can be taken in tea form which is the best for treating this particular ailment. If you're not keen on the tea, you can also choose to inhale the steam of the boiled dried leaves instead. In doing so, you'll help loosen up the mucus in your chest so you can cough them up later.

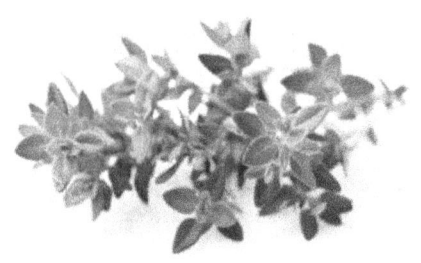

Licorice Root

This contains a compound that has been proven to have very potent antiviral effects against various diseases including the common cold and flu. It can help treat the problem whilst boosting the person's immune system to prevent the cold from coming back. However, when buying these in tea form, do make sure that you're getting actual licorice and not something that only tastes like it. Also, do note that licorice can interact with prescription medicine so do make sure that you speak with your physician before using it.

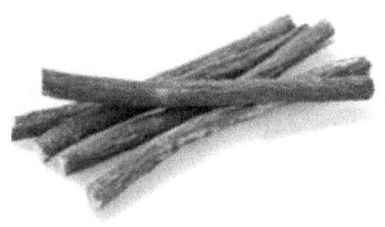

Garlic

This herb helps in boosting the immune system as well as ward off different viruses such as the rhinovirus and the flu. Luckily, these also come in capsule form which should help ease the aroma associated with it. If you're not keen on chewing on a clove of garlic at least twice a day, the supplements would be the next best alternative. Some people also take garlic tea when they have a cold, it can help clear the sinuses and have you back on your feet in a jiffy. Adding a bit of honey to the concoction should tone down the overpowering flavor.

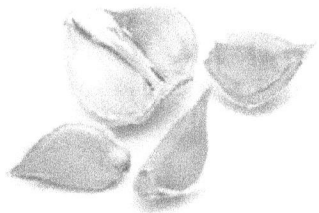

Elderberry Extract

This particular botanical can help with relieving the symptoms of both the cold and the flu. It can help shorten the duration of the symptoms by at least 4 days and because it has antiviral properties, it can prevent both problems from coming back. The berries are commonly taken in tea form, though there are also liquid supplements available which contain its extract.

Honey

Because of its antibacterial and antiviral properties, honey can certainly help when it comes to dealing with the symptoms associated with the cold and the flu. It also helps with the uncomfortable scratchiness one feels in the throat. This can be taken in tea form or as it is. A tablespoon once or twice a day should help get things rolling.

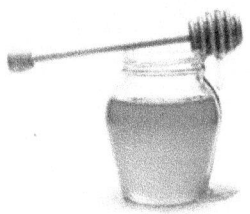

Ginger root

This can be used to treat cold as well as flu-like symptoms along with any headaches that may accompany it. Because of its warming nature, it can stimulate the body and make it produce sweat which then releases toxins and pathogens from the inside. It can also boost the immune system which then shortens the duration of the symptoms as well. It is best taken in tea form.

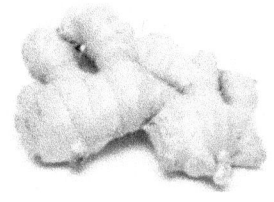

Chapter 4: Remedies for Inflammation

Pain and inflammation can certain put a damper on any fun day you might be having with family and friends. It can also make working difficult and in the end, you're unable to fully focus because of it. People who experience chronic pain are also more prone to developing different psychiatric symptoms such as anxiety and depression.

Fortunately, there are prescription and over-the-counter medicines which are meant to provide relief and help ease the pain. However, they are not the best long term solutions for the issue and taking them regularly can be damaging to the body as a whole. So what can be done in this case? Go natural, of course. There are plenty of herb supplements that can provide the same amount of relief but without leaving any long term effects. Shall we take a closer look?

Capsaicin

This component can be derived from hot chili peppers and is very potent when it comes to treating pain and inflammation. What it does is deplete the P substance which is basically the cause of the pain itself. Capsaicin can be taken as a supplement in pill form but you also have the option of including it in your daily diet by simply adding more hot chili peppers to your dishes.

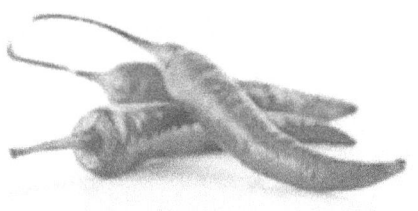

Turmeric

Studies show that the anti-inflammatory properties of turmeric is actually comparable to certain medications like Hydrocortisone and Motrin but without any of the side effects usually associated with both. However, do note that this herb is not recommended for pregnant women as well as individuals who may have any existing gallstone problems. Proper dosage is also important to so do speak to your herbalist or doctor about it.

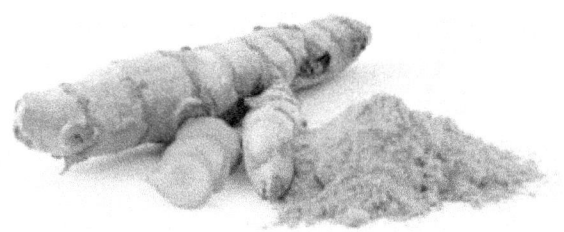

Basil

This fragrant herb that's usually used as a garnish for salads and pastas can actually deliver quite a potent solution for inflammation. It can inhibit the enzyme that causes the problem, very much like what Ibuprofen and Tylenol does for the body. The only difference is that it tastes better and carries with it very little risk of organ damage.

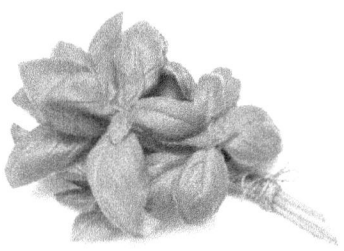

Boswellia

In Ayurvedic medicine, this is commonly used when it comes to treating joint pain and relieving any inflammation associated with it. It works because the herb contains components that are able to eliminate cytokine, the very thing that causes chronic inflammation. There is a risk of developing skin rash after using it, however, so do talk to your physician about the proper way of taking it.

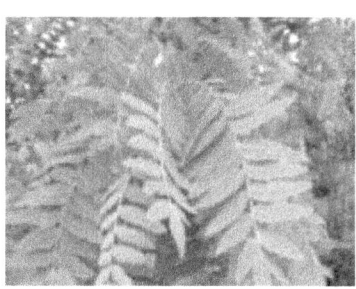

Cinnamon

Who doesn't love the aroma and taste of cinnamon? Add it to your coffee and any kind of pastry you can think of because it has a number of health benefits you'll certain enjoy. Among the benefits would be its ability to help reduce the body's inflammatory responses. It can also ease the pain that goes along with it. Do note that cinnamon can be quite spicy so be sure to take it moderately.

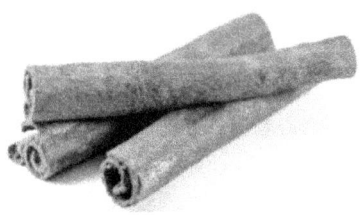

Guggul

Used in Ayurvedic medicine as a means of detoxifying the body, the potency of this herb when it comes to relieving pain as well as inflammation is actually comparable to that of Ibuprofen. Guggul can also help improve certain conditions such as knee osteoarthritis within a couple months of continuous use. The only thing that must be noted when it comes to this botanical would be the fact that it has blood-thinning properties so do avoid taking it together with other similar acting medications.

Chapter 5: Remedies for Menopause Symptoms

Menopause symptoms can be difficult to deal with for a lot of women who are going through it. Some report experiencing hot flashes as significant changes in their moods. There are those who experience sweating and chills regardless of the hour. These things can be experienced by women who are in the pre-menopausal stages as well as those who are "officially" in menopause.

Now, there are many different "treatments" for it. Medication and lifestyle changes are typically recommended to help cope with the uncomfortable symptoms. However, it isn't always easy and note everyone is willing to take medication for the problem.
Luckily, there are herbal alternatives that could help with this problem.

Soy

The isoflavones contained in soy foods aid when it comes to balancing hormone levels and the body. It can also help stimulate estrogen activity. Whilst there are soy supplements readily available in the market, studies show that the best way of getting isoflavones would be through natural soy foods. From tofu, tempeh to soy milk, there's plenty of soy based food to choose from.

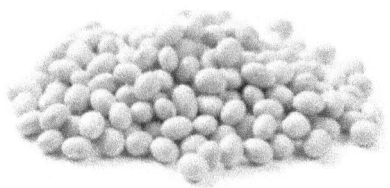

Flaxseed

This contains a component called lignin which is very important when it comes to modulating hormone metabolism. Preparing the seeds is pretty easy as well. Just grab a grinder and make about 1 to 2 tablespoons of it every day.

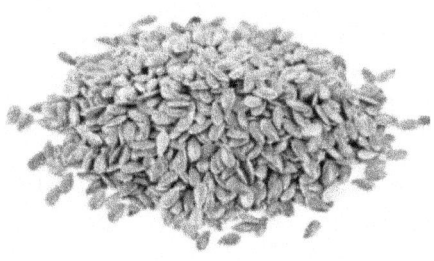

Dong Quai

This is often used in both the West and China when it comes to supporting as well as maintaining the balance of female hormones in the body. However, it does not promote estrogenic activity. Do note that if the woman is experiencing heavy bleeding due to menopause, taking this particular herb is not recommended.

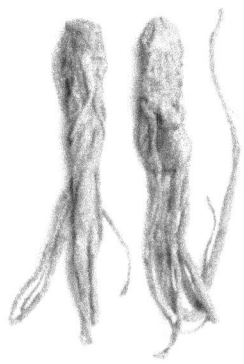

Black Cohosh

If you're looking for something to alleviate the more uncomfortable symptoms of menopause such as hot flashes then this is what you'll need. It works by balancing and maintaining hormonal levels which helps in reducing the severity of the hot flashes. The only thing about it is that, there have been reports of women saying that its effects aren't the same for everyone. It can be more effective for other people and the reason for this is still unknown.

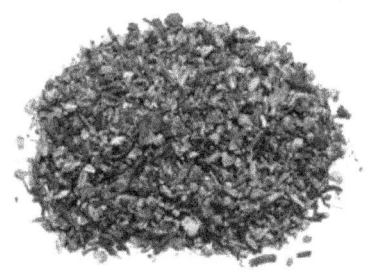

Vitamin E

Daily doses of this will not only help make your skin better and detoxify the body, it can also help with alleviating the effects of hot flashes in menopausal women.

Evening Primrose

During and even after going through menopause, most women would experience dry skin, hair loss, eczema, painful breasts and a much slower healing process which is caused by the lower levels of estrogen in their bodies. Evening primrose is capable of easing all of these symptoms, helping make the process much easier and manageable.

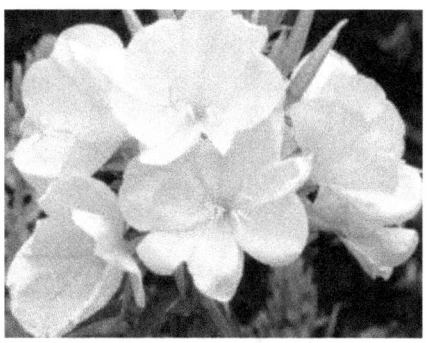

Chapter 6: Remedies for Skin Problems

When it comes to skin problems, natural is always better. After all, the skin can be quite sensitive and needs something gentler when it comes to treating it. Of course, there's also the fact that herbal remedies have little to no side effects so there's no real worry of damaging your skin when using them.

Arnica Flower

When it comes to healing wounds, this botanical is certainly one of the best. It is also used as an analgesic, an anti-inflammatory cream as well as an antiseptic. If you have any swelling or bruises whether it be due to an injury or even surgery, it can help speed up the healing process.

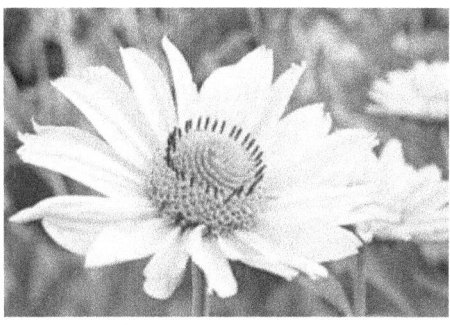

Calendula Flower

In treating skin infections, burns, rashes, bruises and even cuts, this is one of the best botanicals to use. Its use for topical treatments is actually approved by some health authorities. If you have lesions in your mouth, tea can also be made from it which should help alleviate the pain as well as reduce any significant swelling in the affected areas.

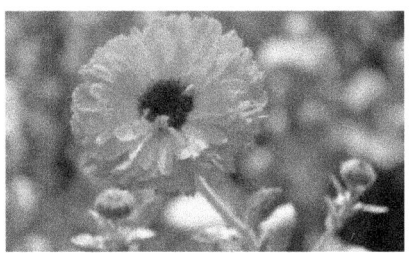

Comfrey

This is very effective when it comes to speeding up the healing process of cuts and bruises. For rashes, it serves as an anti-inflammatory which helps the itchiness, swelling as well as the redness of the affected area. It can also be used for insect bites and any fungal infections on the body. However, it should only be used topically and never ingested. So do avoid using it near your mouth area.

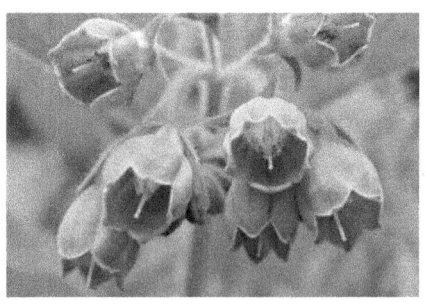

Chamomile

For treating mild skin problems ranging from hives, itchy lesions and sunburn, chamomile is the best. It can even be used as a kind of oral rinse in order to treat any painful mouth lesions that you have.

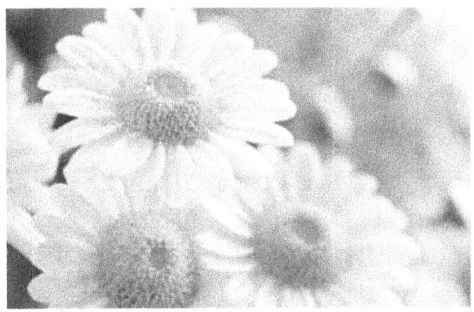

Honey

This is great if you have parts of your skin that's very itchy and red. Honey has soothing effects that would alleviate both while protecting your skin from any infections as well. However, do note that there are people who might be allergic to the product so consult with your doctor or make sure you're not allergic to it before using. Honey can also be used to soothe painful sunburn as well as minor burns.

Witch Hazel

For skin issues such as acne, this can be used as an astringent. It helps dry out the affected area and reduces both swelling as well as the redness. Because it's anti-bacterial, it is also capable of killing off the source of the acne itself.

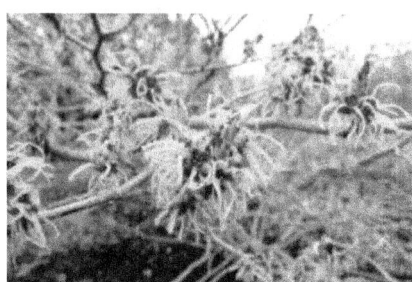

Lavender and Thyme oil mix

These are great for treating alopecia. One only needs to apply it to the affected area topically, massaging until it gets absorbed. It should begin working a month into the first time it was used. However, it needs to be applied on a daily basis.

Potatoes

These contain starch-based compounds which help soothe and reduce the effects of sunburn. All you need to do is chopped an uncooked one and pat one of the slices onto the affected area. You can also choose to grate and chill the potato first before application.

Cucumbers

Because of its cooling effect, placing slices of this on top of your sunburn can help relieve some of the pain as well as swelling if there's any. It can also be turned into a paste to make the application much easier to do.

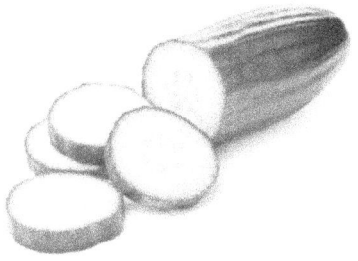

Green Tea

This contains tannic acid as well as catechin which are both great for relieving the pain of sunburn and speeding up the healing process of the skin. Just soak a couple of tea bags in chilled water before applying it like a cold compress onto the affected areas. You can also use the tea extract to wash your face if there's some sunburnt areas upon it as well.

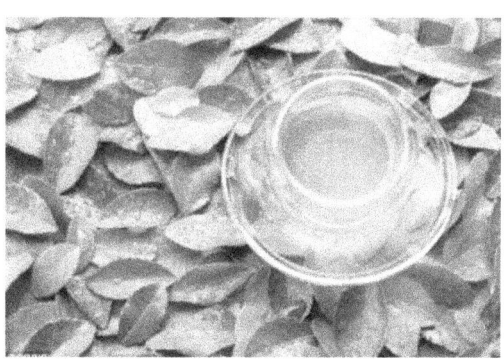

Chapter 7: Natural Remedies for an Upset Stomach

There are plenty of over-the-counter medicines that would help relieve an upset stomach. However, taking these regularly might be causing more damage than you'd like. In fact, some medicines can be so strong that if used constantly, they can start to create problems in the stomach lining. Would you keep on using them if that was the case?

Fortunately, there are natural alternatives. These are far gentler, more affordable and you can take them as often as you'd like without needing to worry about damaging your body.

Mint

Fresh mint can easily soothe an upset stomach especially if you take it in tea form. You can also chew on a mint leaf that works just as well. There are also peppermint supplements available if you're looking for a quicker option. However, buying mint candies might not be a great idea if you're looking to treat an upset stomach. Most of the time, these will contain and sugar which could worsen the problem.

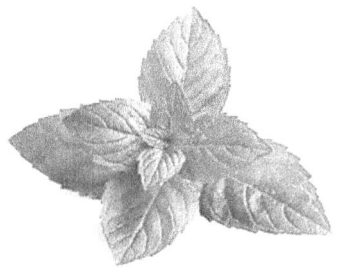

Fennel

Chewing on a fresh slice of its bulb can help ease bloating and digestion especially after a big meal. It can also be taken in tea form. This should help soothe an upset stomach. There are no known side effects to it so you may drink as needed.

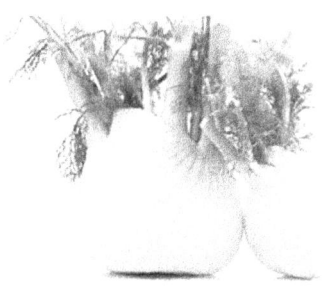

Lemon Water

Lemon is one of the most versatile fruits you can have at home. But as treatment for an upset stomach? Most people would assume that it can worsen it because of its acidity. However, this is not the case. Lemon is actually alkaline so if you're experiencing acidity, having a drink of water infused with it is the best remedy. Just squeeze one into a warm mug of water or drink it slightly cold.

Warm Saltwater

It used to be that saltwater is only taken when it comes to soothing sore throat. However, it can also work wonders on an upset stomach. All you'll need is a cup of warm water as well as a teaspoon of salt. Do drink it as soon as you've prepared it for best results. Do note that if you have high blood pressure or any other health issue that can be triggered by salt, avoid doing this.

Baking Soda

Before you reach for the Alka-Seltzer to ease indigestion and heartburn, try taking baking soda first. It is essentially the exact same thing. All you need to do is mix a teaspoon of it with a warm cup of water.

Aloe Vera Juice

This particular botanical can be used in a number of different ways. There are many benefits to taking it and among those, its ability to soothe and treat various intestinal problems. It is most commonly used for constipation as well as relieving the pains of an upset stomach. Other uses include: bloating, diarrhea, gas and cramps.

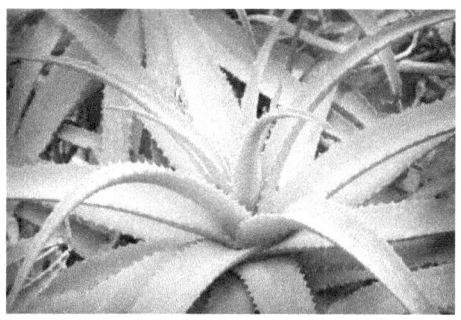

Apple Cider Vinegar

Experiencing indigestion? A few teaspoons of this mixed with some warm water should help relieve that. It can also aid the body when it comes to absorbing nutrients better as well as soothe the pain of hyperacidity. Do make sure that you're using natural and pure apple cider vinegar because any other variety will give you different results.

Conclusion

Thank you again for purchasing this book!

I hope this book was able to help you learn more about Natural remedies!

The next step is to put this information to use and try using some of these natural cures for yourself as well as your family.

Finally, if you enjoyed this book, please take the time to share your thoughts and post a review on Amazon.   It'd be greatly appreciated!

Thank you and good luck!

Bonus Content

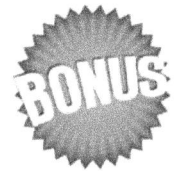

As a token of our appreciation Grand Reveur Publications would like to give you access to our exclusive bonus content (including free eBooks!).

Exclusive pre-release access to our latest eBooks Free Grand Reveur eBooks during promotional periods.

A method ANYONE can use to publish their own book and make passive income

To receive this bonus content visit the following web site:

https://ignorelimits.leadpages.net/grandreveur publications/

As this is a limited time offer it would be a shame to miss out, I recommend grabbing these bonuses before reading on.

www.ingramcontent.com/pod-product-compliance
Lightning Source LLC
Chambersburg PA
CBHW070511290526
45790CB00003B/1195